BELONGS TO CHRISTINE W

Ketogenic Diet: The Keto Diet Guide for Beginners

The Smart and Healthy Way to Lose Weight and Feel Increased Energy

---

With delicious recipes and meal plans

Table of Contents

Conclusion

Introduction

Thank you for purchasing this book, 'Ketogenic Diet: The Keto Diet Guide for Beginners: The smart and healthy way to lose weight and feel increased energy, with delicious recipes and meal plans.

I hope you have an enjoyable and informative read on the ketogenic diet and get to try the recipes as soon you have finished reading the book!

The ketogenic diet has been garnering massive amounts of attention worldwide and you are about to discover why. Not only does it provide you with a lot of benefits, but it also helps you live in a fitter body and maintain a healthy lifestyle, something that everyone is trying to achieve in the present day and age.

This book has detailed the basics of the ketogenic diet, explained how it affects your body, and detailed the many ways your body is going to benefit from it together with giving tips on how to get started on your ketogenic journey.

I wish you luck with leading a fit life in a healthy body!

Thank you.

Chapter 1: What Is The Ketogenic Diet?

To describe it in the easiest way, the ketogenic diet is a diet that has a low content of carbs and high content in fats. That is how it also came about to be named the LCHF die – low carb, high fat.

If we delve a little deeper, the ketogenic diet is instrumental in making your liver produce ketones. What this does is that it shifts your body's focus from making use of glucose in order to fuel itself and instead, turns fat into the main source of power.

When you are on a ketogenic diet, the most basic expectation of you is to completely restrict your consumption of carbohydrates. It takes only a small amount of effort and consideration to make these alterations in your body, and in turn be rewarded by a fitter body and lifestyle.

When it comes to protein or fat, you are allowed to consume just about any amount of both, but it depends on the goals you want to achieve from being on this diet.

Carbs are the key element here. When you maintain a strong hold over your consumption of carbohydrates, this builds or collapses your ketogenic diet. In fact, the presence or the lack thereof of carbs in your food intake is what brands your diet as keto or not.

Metabolism and Hormones

Now that you have been briefed about the ketogenic diet let us have a look at how it affects two very important aspects of your body – your metabolism and your hormones. How a diet affects either can largely impact the quality of your lifestyle as in the case of a diet failing, it could leave you with a set of side-effects or no-effects and if you put all your effort into a diet that does not reward you in any manner, it becomes very demoralizing to consider going on a diet again even if the next diet could have been very beneficial to you because you just won't feel that kind of dedication anymore. So, read on to find out why this diet works.

Keto and Metabolism

Fats, carbohydrates and proteins are what someone's regular diet generally consists of. But as we restrict our intake of carbs and the body is deprived of it, the reserves of energy in our body face quick depletion. And that leads to the body searching for other places to draw its energy from.

That's where fats come in handy. They are a viable alternative for your body to get its required power from – fats that are stored up in your body but under the disposition of acids.

Almost immediately after the energy reserves have depleted, these fats or these acids start getting used by your tissues in order to charge the body. This is how fats become the apex source of your body's energy.

But it is worth mentioning that not all of your organs can make use of these specific fatty acids and that is why ketone bodies or ketones are used.

Ketone bodies are a by-product of the gathering of fatty acids in your liver when they go through a breakdown, albeit a partial one.

When we restrict and deprive our bodies of carbs, this leads to the generation of more ketone bodies that are released into the bloodstream. And that is when **ketosis**, the metabolic state, happens.

When the body starts using ketone bodies to charge up your energy, it faces a decrease in its regular dependency on glucose and, in turn, there is a reduction in the creation and utilization of glucose.

When ketosis takes place, your body lowers the amount of protein in your body so that it can provide you with energy. In fact, a lot of people turn to the ketogenic diet as an effective diet for weight-loss, as it helps remove body fat and simultaneously helps build a body that is lean by acquiring just the right amount of mass.

Keto and Hormones

There are a set of hormonal changes that take place when you do the ketogenic diet – it especially affects the two hormones called insulin and glucagon.

Insulin is the hormone that works as a form of storage hormone. It is instrumental in carrying the nutrients present in your bloodstream directly into your tissues that require these nutrients. It also helps the body store a type of glucose, called glycogen, in the muscles; while the hormone stimulating the body to break down the glycogen that the muscles have stored is called glucagon. It primarily helps in breaking down the glycogen amassed in your liver, to provide you with an ample amount of glucose for the body to work with.

When there is an increase in your glucagon levels, your levels of insulin will start decreasing, as a result of stopping your intake of carbs, which then leads to a quick rise in fatty acids released by your body, which then undergo a breakdown by the liver. This process helps generate ketones and that results in **ketosis**, the metabolic state mentioned earlier.

However, it is worthy to note that there do exist many different hormones that are impacted by this process, but insulin and glucagon are the ones that help shift the body's focus from carbohydrates to fats.

Benefits of the Keto diet

The ketogenic gained its massive popularity owing it to its innumerable health benefits. Some of these are:

Losing Weight

For most people, weight-loss is that one aspect of the keto diet that they are most attracted to and for many, initially, it is the only reason they take up the keto diet. And this is because when we reduce our intake of carbohydrates, it becomes one of the easiest ways to lose weight. Being on a diet that is low in carbs, your body loses the excess amount of water that's present in your body; this lowers our levels of insulin, which means losing the excess sodium from the body. This leads to quick loss of weight. However, after one point, the weight loss slows down to an extent, all for the right reasons. The ketogenic diet makes your weight experience a sheer drop, then makes sure it turns into a steady ongoing process. This is helpful in maintaining your weight loss over a long period of time, given that you follow the diet properly.

Reduced Appetite

The ketogenic focuses on eating a lot of proteins and since proteins tend to be so fulfilling, it eliminates the chances of being hungry as often as you used to be prior to starting this diet. Contrary to what you might think, it boosts your levels of energy and increases your overall capacity of performing everyday tasks.

Reduced Blood Sugar levels

When you are on the keto diet, your body undergoes a series of chemical changes that can act as a barrier between you and Type 2 Diabetes. And if you are already suffering from it, you can get your insulin levels under control by going for this diet.

Foods to eat and avoid

To eat

Meat: steak, turkey, ham, chicken, bacon, sausage and red meat

Fish: tuna, trout, mackerel, salmon or any fish that contains high amounts of natural fats

Eggs: go for pastured eggs since they are rich in omega-3, which adds value to the diet

Butter: grass fed butter

Cream and cheese: blue cheese, cream cheese, goat cheese, mozzarella cheddar cheese – and any cheese that is unprocessed

Vegetables: chives, onions, tomatoes, peppers, lettuce, celery, broccoli, spinach, radishes, cucumber, bok choy, asparagus, endive, zucchini, etc.

Fruits: avocado, and for occasional intake - raspberries, strawberries, blueberries, cranberries, mulberries and coconut.

Nuts and seeds: chia seeds, pumpkin seeds, almonds, walnuts and flaxseeds

Healthy oils: extra virgin olive oil, avocado oil, coconut oil

Condiments: Salt, herbs, pepper, mayonnaise, lemon juice, lime zest, etc.

To avoid

Root vegetables and tubers: carrots, potatoes, sweet potatoes, parsnips

Beans and legumes: lentils, peas, chickpeas and kidney beans

Grains and cereals: rice, pasta, wheat products, breads

Fruits: anything rich in sugar – mangoes, apples, etc.

Chapter 2: How to Get Started

With like any other diet, a bit of preparation or having a basic idea on how to approach the technicalities can go a very long way. Some helpful tips have been outlined for you to help you get started with your ketogenic diet.

As compared to most diets, the ketogenic diet is far easier to follow, as it does not have a lot of restrictions except the exclusion or bare inclusion of carbs in the diet.

Pantry cleansing

Getting any possible distractions or obstacles out of your diet's way is always the smart thing to do. For this, you need to begin with your pantry, which is going to lay the very foundation of your diet.

Remove anything that is not compatible with the keto diet. As you have already been briefed about the dietary dos and don'ts of this diet, you are by now aware of the foods that should or should not be within your grasp.

Start by removing food products that are processed or considered junk. Remove the junk and then the carbs.

Keep in mind that the ketogenic diet demands of you to consume carbohydrates in really small quantities, so, it is essential you rid yourself of any heavy carbohydrates within sight.

Next, pick out the food rich in sugar, or which are sugary in any manner! They are nothing but just more carbohydrates. Next up, packaged foods need to be removed. They are a mountain of preservatives, artificial sweeteners and other added ingredients.

If you are wondering why is this step necessary – well, it is to ensure you do not deviate from the diet you are going to put your time, energy and efforts into. Also, by 'cleansing' this doesn't mean throwing everything away. Instead of letting all of those ingredients go to waste, you can simply donate them at NGOs and soup kitchens. For any cooked dishes that are good and fresh, you could have some friends over finish it up.

Time to shop!

Once you have successfully cleansed your pantry, the next logical thing to do is stock it with keto friendly ingredients. What this helps ensure is that once you have stocked up on all the ingredients required to start off on this diet – it works as a good motivation to stay on track, because you will not want all of those ingredients to go to waste or sit rotting in your pantry.

Read before you buy

When you are out shopping for groceries, make sure an ample amount of your focus goes into reading the labels and not just the price. First, be firm in your resolve to not buy anything that is not a part of your diet, because if it is not adding value to the diet, it is not worth buying.

It is essential you make it a habit of being aware of the labels and reading them and especially the nutrition section before you even consider buying the item in question. It is the norm to pay more attention to quality and price, but when you are on the ketogenic diet, you could be undoing it all by 'accidentally' buying ingredients that could render all your efforts useless.

The fruit juice you added to your cart may not be giving you all the healthy goodness you thought. Read the nutrition section; it is most likely loaded with sugar. Also, do not fall for so called 'low-fat diet food' products. They're just trouble.

Processed and packaged foods were mentioned earlier to be removed from your pantry simply because they are storehouses of carbohydrates and added sugars. It is only when you make an active effort to see or read the information on food products do you realize what harmful things you have been putting into your body.

So, be sure to read the labels before buying. This will help ensure you stay within the guidelines of the diet.

Bulk Buying

It is natural for you to feel a little rebellious towards change when you venture into any kind of diet. There will be external distractions and internal objections. Temptations will try to lure you into deviating from the diet you are working so hard to maintain. In fact, the initial days of any diet can be really bothersome because you instantly start craving any food you have loved all your life, but have to stay away from because of the diet. This is an issue that needs to be addressed with care. Deviating in the very first week can be very demoralizing and might even not let you return to the diet.

Once you are beyond this stage, it becomes way easier to stick to the diet for as long as possible – preferably a lifetime.

And to help you with this here's one of the greatest tips – buy in bulk.

Buy your groceries in bulk when you do that, you are benefiting from it in three ways:

- You save a lot of money because larger packets cost less.
- You save a lot of time, buying in bulk means fewer trips to the grocery store or supermarket.

- It stops you from deviating. Stocking up your pantry in bulk with all your required groceries ensures you don't deviate from the diet. This is because there is no way one would want to let all those ingredients and foods to go waste. Just because you saved some money while buying everything does not mean you want what you spent on your groceries to go to waste. In fact, groceries become a reason to stick to the diet instead of being an excuse to deviate from it in case you find you don't have enough groceries. You will also find that you are more prone to eating out if you don't have the necessary food at home. This is why a pantry that has been stocked up properly can play such a huge role in motivating you when you are on the ketogenic diet.

No Eating Out Before Beginning the Diet

It has become the norm to eat out as frequently as possible. Regularly eating home cooked meals has almost become a thing of the past. It might be a social thing or something put into place by other factors, but the point is – we do not even realize how much we are harming our bodies by constantly eating out. This frequency is, in fact, something that could dissuade you when you are trying to stick to a diet; which is why it is important you restrict eating out completely before you start the diet.

An entire chapter has been dedicated to tips to eating out when on keto, but be sure to keep in mind that it helps a lot to quit eating out before you start the diet, because the initial stage of any diet is its most crucial – and if you can reign in your urges in the days before you start the diet and the first initial weeks – you will only end up amplifying the benefits of this diet. So bear in mind to reduce how often you are eating out before starting your keto diet.

Minimal Consumption of Root Vegetables

As you might have noticed from the section on what to or not to eat during the ketogenic diet, there is hardly any limitation on the intake of fruit and vegetables. However, it is essential you are aware of your consumption of root veggies. The reason behind this is because they are full of carbohydrates and sugars. The sole intent behind the diet is to minimize your intake of carbohydrates to very small quantities. Even if you buy these root vegetables, buy them in really small quantities. Another aspect of them worthy of noting is the presence of starch in most of these – and starch is nothing but more carbs on your plate. Thus, be very careful around these kinds of vegetables that are nothing but invited trouble should you wish to indulge in them.

Three Step Prepping

Do not rush into the ketogenic diet. It is always better to take some time and properly plan it out and if you do want to get the best out of it -

Prepare

Prepare yourself for the oncoming changes. People find change or any alteration in their routine to be disorienting. Just like that, making changes in your diet could affect you in many ways – be it physically or mentally. And that is why it is of utmost importance to properly prepare yourself for these changes. Once you know that you really do want to do the diet – there will be nothing to stop you. The dedication you put into your diet will reward you with a healthy body, fitter mind, and a great health oriented lifestyle.

Plan it out

Composing a plan beforehand helps build an outline for you to work with. This way, you do not deviate from the goals you have set for yourself when on the diet. It is important for you to take certain steps such as making grocery lists to buy your keto essentials and ingredients. And when you are out buying those ingredients, read the labels! The nutritional information on the labels can make or break your diet.

Plan other important things as well – like your meal times, and remind yourself to drink lots of water.

Schedule your carbs

As weird as it might sound, tricking your body into assuming there has been no consumption of carbs is kind of easy. To know when to schedule your carbs is a significant aspect of the keto diet. In fact, one of the best times to consume carbohydrates is prior to your work out regime.

Chapter 3: Tips on Eating Out While On Keto

In the previous chapter, it was advised to restrict eating out when you are about to start your keto diet. If the prospect of never eating out scared you – don't worry!

Once you have started on your diet, and everything is going steady, you can eat out but with a few guidelines kept in mind. Just because you are on a diet should not mean you will give up on your social life; and let's face it – the majority of our social gatherings involve food!

So, here's how you can save yourself from getting off track with the diet, given that you stick to the guideline if you really do want to get the best results from the diet.

Say No to Starch

Skip the pasta, bounce the potatoes, and turn away from the bread and rice. There will be no temptations if distracting and tempting items do not make an appearance on your plate. Avoid ordering starchy foods to avoid consuming them. Yes, it is not as easy as it sounds.

If you order a burger or a sandwich, ask the restaurant if they can replace the bun with lettuce wraps. A lot of restaurants do this. When you order an entrée, ask the restaurant to substitute the starch with extra vegetables or a salad. And in case they refuse to substitute, just remove the unnecessary item, anyway.

But if despite ordering carefully, you are served a plate with some starchy side, think about the options available to you. If you feel confident, you can let the starchy be, let it exist on your plate untouched – great. But if there's even the tiniest threat of you having even a bite – instantly ask the server to re-plate the dish you were served but with the exclusion of the starch. And if at a casual setting – discard the unwanted starch from your plate straight into the trash.

If there is any awkwardness or if you think you think or feel you need to explain yourself – be it to the waiter or whoever you are dining with – do so by mentioning a diet that is restrictive or tummy issues.

Include healthy fats

A majority of the meals served in restaurants tend to be low on their fat content, and this makes it difficult to feel full on such food if you have excluded carbs from the meal, however, there is a way to fix this problem.

Ask for vinegar and olive oil dressing then liberally drizzle the oil on your meal or salads.

Butter makes it better. Stick true to this saying by asking for some extra butter to melt on your meat or veggies.

You can even arm yourself with olive oil by carrying it in a tiny bottle as a lot of low-carb veterans do. The reason behind this is that restaurants serve vegetable oils of a cheaper variety (they are high on omega 6 fat) instead of olive oil – and that can be rather unhealthy. To avoid such scenarios, simply carry some with you.

Dessert

Ask yourself if you still are hungry. If you are not, then you can opt for a cup of tea or coffee while you wait on others to be done with their dessert. You can also opt for herbal tea or decaf, in case it's late.

And if you are indeed still hungry and need a few more bites of food, check if it is possible to order a plate of berries with some heavy cream or even if a plate of cheese would be available.

If you go the coffee way, try adding some butter or cream to add a 'filling' factor.

When visiting friends or family

Consider communicating your dietary preferences prior to the gathering, so that it gives the host some time to accommodate your preferences.

If there is a need for you to explain yourself – tummy issues or restrictive diet are your go-to excuse.

You can also choose to snack on something fatty to partially fill you up before you leave home; cheese, nuts, olives – any keto friendly bite-able snack to munch on.

Another smart thing to do in such scenarios is to pick something at the party and indulge a bit in it since such occasions are usually just for a meal – it is a very okay thing to do. Say, indulge in the fried chicken's crispy fried coating. Small things can go a long way – it will also cheer your spirits up.

Chapter 4: Ketogenic Breakfast Recipes

Ultimate Breakfast Roll Ups

Serves: 4

Ingredients:

- 8 large eggs
- 1 1/3 cups cheddar cheese, shredded
- 4 breakfast sausage patties, cooked
- Salt to taste
- Pepper to taste
- 4 slices bacon, cooked
- Cooking spray

Method:

1. Place a nonstick skillet over medium high heat. Spray with cooking spray. When the pan heats, lower heat to medium low.
2. Add 2 eggs into a bowl and whisk well. Add salt and pepper and whisk well.
3. Pour into the skillet. Cover the skillet and cook until eggs are nearly done. Carefully slide the egg on a plate. Spread 1/3-cup cheese all over the wrap.
4. Place a strip of bacon. Cut a sausage patty into 2 pieces and place on the wrap. Roll and place with its seam side facing down. Serve.

5. Repeat all the above 4 steps and make the remaining roll ups.

3 Cheese Quiche Stuffed Peppers

Serves: 2

Ingredients:

- 1 medium bell pepper, halved lengthwise, deseeded
- ¼ cup ricotta cheese
- ¼ cup parmesan cheese, grated + 2 tablespoons extra to garnish
- ¼ cup mozzarella cheese, shredded
- 2 large eggs
- A large handful baby spinach leaves
- ¼ teaspoon dried parsley
- ½ teaspoon garlic powder

Method:

1. Add all the cheeses, garlic powder, eggs and parsley into the food processor bowl. Process until well combined.
2. Fill this mixture into the pepper halves. Do not fill up to the top.
3. Place spinach leaves on top. Push the leaves into the mixture.
4. Cover each bell pepper with foil.
5. Bake in a preheated oven at 375° F until cooked.
6. Unwrap and sprinkle Parmesan cheese on top. Broil for a few minutes until light brown on top.

Spinach Herb and Feta Wraps

Serves: 4

Ingredients:

- 6 egg whites
- 10 whole eggs
- 2 teaspoons sesame oil
- 1 teaspoon salt
- Pepper to taste
- 1 cup feta cheese, crumbled
- 6 whole sundried tomatoes, chopped
- 4 cups spinach leaves
- 8 basil leaves, roughly chopped
- 2 teaspoons olive oil (optional)

Method:

1. Place a nonstick skillet over medium high heat. Spray with cooking spray. When the pan heats, lower heat to medium low.
2. Add eggs, whites and sesame oil into a bowl and whisk well. Add salt and pepper and whisk well.
3. Pour ¼ of the egg mixture into the skillet. Cover the skillet and cook until eggs are nearly done. Carefully slide the egg on a plate.
4. Repeat the above 3 steps to make the remaining 3 wraps.

5. To make filling: Place the skillet back over heat. Add spinach and sauté for a minute or 2 until the spinach wilts. Turn off the heat.
6. Place the wraps on a serving platter. Divide and layer the wraps with spinach, feta cheese and basil. Drizzle ½ teaspoon olive oil all over each wrap if using.
7. Wrap and place with its seam side facing down.
8. Serve.

Mini Pancake Donuts

Serves: 11

Ingredients:

- 1.5 ounces cream cheese
- 2 tablespoons almond flour
- 2 medium eggs
- ½ tablespoon coconut flour
- ½ teaspoon vanilla extract
- ½ teaspoon baking powder
- 5 drops liquid stevia
- 2 tablespoons erythritol

Method:

1. Add all the ingredients into a bowl and blend with an immersion blender until smooth.
2. Preheat a mini donut maker. Spray the donut cavities with coconut oil.
3. Spoon batter into each cavity. Cook for 3 minutes. Flip sides and cook the other side for 2 minutes.
4. Remove from the donut maker and serve.
5. Repeat the above steps with the remaining batter, if any.

Avocado Bacon Muffins

Serves: 8

Ingredients:

- 3 medium eggs
- 1 tablespoon butter
- 2 ½ slices bacon
- 2 tablespoons flaxseed meal
- ¼ cup almond flour
- 2 teaspoons psyllium husk powder
- 2 ¼ ounces Colby Jack cheese, grated
- 1 medium avocado, peeled, pitted, chopped into small pieces
- 2 small spring onions, chopped
- ½ teaspoon dried chives
- ½ teaspoon dried cilantro
- ½ teaspoon garlic, minced
- Red chili flakes to taste
- Pepper to taste
- Salt to taste
- 2 teaspoons lemon juice
- ¾ cup coconut milk
- ½ teaspoon baking powder

Method:

1. Add eggs, flaxseed meal, almond flour, all the spices, lemon juice and coconut milk into a mixing bowl. Whisk until well combined. Set aside for a while.

2. Place a pan over medium low heat. Add bacon and cook until it is nearly crisp. Add butter. Remove bacon with a slotted spoon and place on a plate. When cool enough to handle, crumble.
3. Add spring onions, cheese, baking powder, bacon and the mixture of butter and fat remaining in the pan into the egg mixture.
4. Add avocado and fold gently.
5. Divide and pour into greased muffin cups.
6. Bake in a preheated oven at 350° F until cooked through. It should take around 25 minutes.

French toast Muffin

Serves: 5-6

Ingredients:

- 3 large eggs
- 2 tablespoons peanut butter
- 1/3 cup almond flour
- 2 tablespoons toasted almonds, crushed
- 2 tablespoons heavy whipping cream
- 1 tablespoon coconut oil
- 1 tablespoon erythritol
- ½ teaspoon vanilla extract
- ½ teaspoon ground cinnamon
- ¼ teaspoon salt
- 5 drops liquid stevia
- 1/8 teaspoon ground nutmeg
- ½ tablespoon butter, unsalted

Method:

1. Add almond flour, cinnamon, erythritol, salt, cinnamon and nutmeg into a bowl and mix well.
2. Add butter, coconut oil and peanut butter into a microwave safe bowl. Microwave for 30-40 seconds or until it melts. Whisk well.
3. Pour into the bowl of almond flour. Mix until well combined.
4. Pour into cupcake trays. Sprinkle almonds on top.

5. Bake in a preheated oven at 350° F until cooked through. It should take around 25 minutes.
6. When done, remove from the oven and cool for a few minutes.
7. Top with a little whipped cream and serve.

Breakfast Stack

Serves: 2

Ingredients:

- 20 slices bacon
- 8 cups spinach
- 4 tablespoons bacon fat
- 8 large eggs
- 4 tablespoons heavy cream
- ½ teaspoon salt or to taste
- 1 cup cheddar cheese, shredded
- ½ tablespoon Mrs. Dash table blend
- ½ teaspoon pepper powder

Method:

1. Take 10 slices bacon and weave it into a 5 x 5 weave. Repeat with the remaining 10 slices to make the other weave.
2. Place in a baking dish.
3. Bake in a preheated oven at 400° F until cooked. Remove the baking dish from the oven and remove the weaves with a slotted spoon. Place the weaves on a plate lined with paper towels.
4. Use 4 tablespoons of the bacon fat that is left behind in the dish (as mentioned in the list of ingredients). Discard the remaining fat or use in some other recipe.

5. Meanwhile, whisk together in a bowl eggs and cream.
6. Place a skillet over medium heat. Add bacon fat. Add spinach and cook until it wilts. Remove spinach and place in a bowl.
7. Place the skillet back over heat. Add egg mixture, salt and pepper. Scramble the eggs.
8. Place a weave each on 2 plates. Divide the scrambled eggs over the weaves.
9. Top with cheese. Broil for a few minutes for 3-4 minutes.
10. Cool for 5 minutes and serve.

Chapter 5: Ketogenic Smoothie Recipes

Berry Smoothie

Serves: 4

Ingredients:

- 2 cups full fat coconut milk
- 4 egg yolks
- 1 1/3 cups frozen berries of your choice
- ¾ cup water
- 2 scoops whey protein powder, unsweetened

Method:

1. Add coconut milk, yolks, berries, water and whey protein powder into a blender and blend until smooth. Add more water if you like a smoothie of thinner consistency.
2. Pour into tall glasses and serve with crushed ice.

Vanilla Smoothie

Serves: 2

Ingredients:

- 4 large egg yolks
- ½ cup water
- 2 tablespoons coconut oil or MCT oil
- 2 tablespoons powdered erythritol or 6 drops stevia
- 1 cup mascarpone cheese
- 8 ice cubes
- 1 teaspoon pure vanilla extract
- Whipped cream to top (optional)

Method:

1. Add all the ingredients into a blender and blend until smooth.
2. Pour into tall glasses. Spoon whipped cream on top and serve.

Frozen Peppermint Hot Chocolate

Serves: 2

Ingredients:

- ¾ cup almond milk, unsweetened
- ¼ cup keto friendly chocolate protein powder, unsweetened
- ½ teaspoon peppermint liquid stevia
- 1.5 ounces dark chocolate, unsweetened
- 1 cup ice cubes
- ¼ teaspoons peppermint extract

Method:

1. Add almond milk, protein powder, stevia, dark chocolate, ice cubes and peppermint extract into a blender and blend until smooth.
2. Pour into tall glasses and serve.

Green Lemon Smoothie

Serves: 2

Ingredients:

- 1 large avocado, peeled, pitted, chopped
- 6 tablespoons lemon juice
- 1 cup coconut milk or coconut cream
- 2 scoops bulletproof collagen protein
- 2 cups ice cubes
- 1 cucumber, chopped
- 4 cups fresh spinach, chopped, lightly steamed
- 2 tablespoons brain octane oil
- 2 scoops bulletproof whey protein
- Xylitol or stevia to taste
- 5-6 drops lemon essential oil

Method:

1. Add all the ingredients into a blender and blend until smooth. Add water if you like a smoothie of thinner consistency.
2. Pour into glasses and serve.

Raspberry Avocado Smoothie

Serves: 4

Ingredients:

- 2 ripe avocados, peeled pitted, chopped
- 6 tablespoons lemon juice
- 1 cup frozen raspberries, unsweetened
- 2/3 cup water
- 1 tablespoon swerve or erythritol or to taste

Method:

1. Add all the ingredients into a blender and blend until smooth. Add water if you like a smoothie of thinner consistency.
2. Pour into glasses and serve.

Mexican Chocolate Shake

Serves: 2

Ingredients:

- ½ cup coconut cream
- 2 tablespoons ground chia seeds
- ½ teaspoon vanilla extract
- ½ teaspoon cayenne pepper
- Ice cubes, as required
- 4 tablespoons extra-virgin coconut oil
- 4 tablespoons cocoa powder, unsweetened
- ½ teaspoon cinnamon powder
- 2 cups water

Method:

1. Add all the ingredients into a blender and blend until smooth. Add water if you like a smoothie of thinner consistency.
2. Pour into glasses and serve.

Pumpkin Smoothie

Serves: 2

Ingredients:

- ½ cup pumpkin puree
- ½ cup vanilla or plain whey protein or egg white protein powder, unsweetened
- ½ cup crème fraiche or sour cream or plain full fat yogurt or coconut milk
- 2 teaspoons erythritol or 5-6 drops stevia
- ½ cup whipped cream or coconut cream to top

Method:

1. Add all the ingredients into a blender and blend until smooth.
2. Pour into tall glasses. Spoon whipped cream on top and serve.

Chapter 6: Ketogenic Snack Recipes

Sesame Crisp Bread

Serves: 15

Ingredients:

- 6 tablespoons sesame seeds
- 1 ounce cheese, shredded
- 3 ½ tablespoons water
- Salt to taste
- 3 tablespoons sunflower seeds
- 2 tablespoons ground psyllium husk powder
- 1 egg

Method:

1. Add all the ingredients into a bowl and mix well.
2. Line a baking sheet with parchment paper. Place the seed mixture on the parchment paper and spread it evenly.
3. Sprinkle sea salt over it. Cut into 15 equal pieces.
4. Bake in a preheated oven at 350° F for 20 minutes. Lower heat to 280° F and bake for 30-40 minutes or until crisp.
5. Serve or store in an airtight container and serve later.

Prosciutto Wrapped Mozzarella

Serves: 12

Ingredients:

- 12 thin slices prosciutto
- 36 mozzarella ciliegine balls
- 36 fresh basil leaves
- Freshly cracked pepper to taste
- Salt to taste

Method:

1. Slice each prosciutto into 1-inch wide strips. It should be nearly the diameter of the mozzarella ball.
2. Place the prosciutto strips on a serving platter, next to each other.
3. Place a leaf of basil at one end of each strip of prosciutto.
4. Place a ball of mozzarella over each leaf. Sprinkle salt and pepper. Roll and serve.

Salad Sandwiches

Serves: 2

Ingredients:

- 6 leaves cosmopolitan lettuce or Romaine hearts
- Cheese slices, as required
- Dried meat, as required
- 1 avocado, peeled, pitted, sliced
- 1 large tomato, sliced

Method:

1. Place 3 lettuce leaves on each serving plate.
2. Place rest of the ingredients over the lettuce leaves.
3. Serve.

Cheese Chips

Serves: 8

Ingredients:

- 1 teaspoon paprika powder
- 16 ounces cheddar cheese or edam cheese or provolone cheese slices

Method:

1. Line a baking sheet with parchment paper. Place cheese slices over it.
2. Dust with paprika powder.
3. Bake in a preheated oven at 400° F for 8-10 minutes, until crisp. Keep a watch over the cheese after 5 minutes of baking so that it does not get burnt.
4. Serve cheese chips with guacamole.

Cheese Meatballs

Serves: 18

Ingredients:

- 2.2 pounds ground beef
- 6 tablespoons parmesan cheese
- 1 teaspoon salt
- 7 ounces mozzarella cheese or cheddar cheese, chopped into 1 cm cubes
- 2 teaspoons garlic powder
- 1 teaspoon pepper powder

Method:

1. Set aside the cheese and add rest of the ingredients into a bowl.
2. Divide the mixture into as many portions as the number of cheese cubes.
3. Make balls of the meat mixture by placing the cheese in the center.
4. Place a nonstick pan over medium flame and add the meatballs in it. Cover with a lid and cook until brown (do not disturb for a while). Turn the balls and cook until the other side is brown.
5. Serve.

Cheese Puffs

Serves: 6

Ingredients:

- 11 ounce Brie cheese, preferably President Brie
- Paprika to taste
- Dried herbs of your choice to taste
- Garlic powder to taste

Method:

1. Remove the rind of the cheese. Chop into ½ inch cubes. Discard the white edge.
2. Place some cubes of cheese on a microwave safe plate that is lined with parchment paper. Cook in batches.
3. Microwave on High for 1-2 minutes. Keep a watch on it as it can burn easily.
4. Cool for a while. Sprinkle paprika, garlic powder and dried herbs on top and serve.

Chapter 7: Ketogenic Salad Recipes

Salad Nicoise

Serves: 4

Ingredients:

For salad:

- 4 eggs, hard boiled, peeled, cubed
- 14 ounces fresh green beans, trimmed, parboiled
- 3-4 cloves garlic, chopped (optional)
- 4 ounces cherry tomatoes
- 2 cans tuna in olive oil
- Salt to taste
- Pepper to taste
- 6 ounces turnip or celery root, cut into ½ inch pieces, parboiled
- 4 tablespoons olive oil
- 14 ounces lettuce or Romaine lettuce, torn
- 1 red onion, chopped
- 4 ounces olives, pitted, sliced

For dressing:

- 1 tablespoon Dijon mustard
- 2 ounces anchovies
- ½ cup keto friendly mayonnaise

- Juice of a lemon
- 4 tablespoons small capers
- 1 cup olive oil
- A handful fresh parsley, chopped
- 2 cloves garlic, minced (optional)

Method:

1. Add all the ingredients of the dressing into a bowl and blend with an immersion blender until smooth and well combined. Cover and set aside for a while for the flavors to set in.
2. Place a skillet over medium high heat. Add oil. When the oil is heated, add green beans and sauté for a couple of minutes.
3. Add garlic and sauté until fragrant. Add salt and pepper. Toss well.
4. Divide the lettuce among 4 plates. Top with rest of the ingredients.
5. Spoon the dressing over it and serve.

Chicken Salad Eggs

Serves: 4

Ingredients:

- 12 eggs, hard boiled, peeled, halved lengthwise
- 4 tablespoons keto friendly mayonnaise
- 1 small onion, chopped
- 1 teaspoon dill
- Old bay seasoning to garnish
- 2 cups chicken, cooked, finely chopped
- 2 teaspoons Dijon mustard
- ¼ teaspoon celery salt
- 1 teaspoon lemon pepper seasoning

Method:

1. Add all the ingredients except eggs into a bowl and mix well. Set aside.
2. Scoop out the yolk from the eggs and add into the salad bowl. Mix well. Set the whites aside.
3. Refrigerate for a while.
4. Stuff this mixture in the cavity of the egg whites. Place some on top, in a heap.
5. Sprinkle old bay seasoning on top and serve.

Caesar Salad

Serves: 4

Ingredients:

- 1 1/3 pounds chicken breasts
- Salt to taste
- Pepper to taste
- 1 bunch Romaine lettuce
- 2 tablespoons olive oil or melted butter
- 11 ounces bacon, cooked until crisp
- 4 ounces parmesan cheese, freshly grated

For dressing:

- 1 cup keto friendly mayonnaise
- Juice of a lemon
- Zest of a lemon, grated
- 4 tablespoons anchovies, finely chopped
- 2 tablespoons Dijon mustard
- 4 tablespoons parmesan cheese, grated
- Salt to taste
- Pepper to taste

Method:

1. Add all the ingredients of the dressing into a bowl and blend with an immersion blender until smooth and well combined. Cover and set aside for a while for the flavors to set in.

2. Grease a baking dish. Place chicken breasts in it. Sprinkle salt and pepper over the chicken. Trickle oil or butter over it.
3. Bake in a preheated oven at 400° F for about 20 minutes or until cooked.
4. Divide the lettuce among 4 plates. Place chicken over it. Top with bacon and Parmesan cheese.
5. Spoon the dressing over it and serve.

Warm Kale Salad

Serves: 2

Ingredients:

- 1 ounce butter
- Salt to taste
- Pepper to taste
- 1 tablespoon keto friendly mayonnaise
- 1 tablespoon olive oil
- 2 ounces blue cheese or feta cheese, crumbled
- 4 ounces kale, discard hard ribs and stems, torn into bite size pieces
- 6 tablespoons heavy whipping cream
- ½ teaspoon Dijon mustard
- 1 small clove garlic, minced

Method:

1. Place a pan over medium flame and add butter. When butter melts, add kale and sauté until it turns bright green in color. Turn off the heat. Transfer into a bowl.
2. Sprinkle salt and pepper.
3. Whisk together rest of the ingredients except cheese into a bowl. Add salt and pepper and whisk well. Pour over the kale.
4. Fold gently. Top with cheese and serve.

Avocado, Bacon and Goat's Cheese Salad

Serves: 2

Ingredients:

- 4 ounces goat's cheese, cut into round ½ inch slices
- 1 avocado, peeled, pitted, chopped
- 2 ounces arugula
- 4 ounces bacon
- 2 ounces walnuts, chopped
- Salt to taste
- Pepper to taste

For dressing:

- 2 tablespoons lemon juice
- ¼ cup olive oil
- ¼ cup keto friendly mayonnaise
- 1 tablespoon heavy whipping cream

Method:

1. To make dressing: Add lemon juice, olive oil, mayonnaise and cream into a bowl and blend with an immersion blender until smooth and well combined. Cover and set aside for a while for the flavors to set in.
2. Line a baking dish with parchment paper. Place the cheese slices in it.
3. Place rack in the upper part of the oven.

4. Bake in a preheated oven at 400° F for until golden brown in color.
5. Meanwhile, place a pan over medium flame and add the bacon and let it become crisp. Remove and set aside. When cool enough to handle, chop into smaller pieces.
6. Divide the arugula between 2 plates. Divide bacon and goat's cheese and place over arugula.
7. Top with walnuts. Sprinkle salt and pepper. Spoon the dressing on top and serve.

Chicken and Berry Summer Salad

Serves: 4

Ingredients:

- 2 chicken breasts, cubed
- 1 ½ cups blueberries
- 12 strawberries, chopped
- 1 cup walnuts, chopped
- 4 cups spinach, torn
- 6 tablespoons raspberry balsamic vinegar
- 1/3 cup feta cheese, crumbled

Method:

1. Place a nonstick pan over medium flame and add chicken and cook until tender.
2. Add the chicken into a large serving bowl. Add blueberries, strawberries, walnuts, and spinach and toss well.
3. Drizzle vinegar on top. Toss well.
4. Divide into 4 plates. Top with crumbled feta cheese and serve right away.

Keto Apple Slaw

Serves: 8

Ingredients:

- 6 cups broccoli slaw
- 2 green onions, chopped
- 4 teaspoons poppy seeds
- 1 teaspoon lemon juice
- ½ cup sour cream
- 2 apples, cored, shredded
- 4 ounces pecans, chopped
- 2 teaspoons apple cider vinegar
- ½ cup keto friendly mayonnaise
- ½ teaspoon salt

Method:

1. Add poppy seeds, lemon juice, mayonnaise, apple cider vinegar and sour cream into a bowl. Whisk until well combined. Set aside for a while for the flavors to set in.
2. Add broccoli slaw into a large bowl. Add apple and mix well.
3. Add green onions and pecans. Toss well.
4. Add the dressing and fold gently. Add salt and fold again.
5. Divide into plates and serve right away.

Chapter 8: Ketogenic Soup Recipes

Broccoli Cheddar Soup

Serves: 4

Ingredients:

- 2 cups broccoli florets
- 1 ¾ cups chicken broth
- 1 ½ cups cheddar cheese, shredded
- 2 cloves garlic, minced
- ½ cup heavy cream
- 1 teaspoon butter
- Salt to taste
- Pepper to taste

Method:

1. Place a soup pot over medium heat. Add butter. When butter melts, garlic and sauté for about a minute until fragrant.
2. Add broth, broccoli and cream and bring to the boil.
3. Lower heat and simmer until broccoli is cooked. Add cheese and stir constantly for a few minutes until cheese melts.
4. Add salt and pepper and stir. Turn off the heat when the cheese melts.
5. Ladle into soup bowls and serve.

High Fat Hamburger Soup

Serves: 3

Ingredients:

- 1 medium red onion, chopped
- 1 medium yellow bell pepper, sliced
- 2 tablespoons red palm oil, melted
- Freshly ground pepper to taste
- 2 cloves garlic, minced
- 2 cups beef stock with fat
- 10 Brussels sprouts, halved
- Himalayan rock salt to taste
- ½ pound grass fed regular ground beef
- 3 stalks celery, chopped
- 1 cup whole tomatoes
- 1 bay leaf
- 1/8 teaspoon cayenne pepper or chili powder
- 5 mushrooms, chopped
- ½ tablespoon tomato paste
- ½ teaspoon dried oregano
- 2 tablespoons fresh parsley, chopped

Method:

1. Place mushrooms, onion, bell pepper, oil, salt, pepper and Brussels sprouts into a bowl and toss well. Spread on a baking sheet.
2. Roast in a preheated oven at 350° F for 25-30 minutes. When done, remove from the oven and set aside.

3. Place a soup pot over medium heat. Add beef and sauté until brown. Break it simultaneously as it cooks. Add celery and garlic and sauté for a couple of minutes until fragrant.
4. Add rest of the ingredients and stir. Bring to the boil.
5. Lower heat and cover with a lid. Simmer for 15-20 minutes.
6. Add the roasted vegetables and heat thoroughly. Garnish with parsley.
7. Ladle into soup bowls and serve with Flax focaccia.

Pumpkin Chipotle Soup

Serves: 3

Ingredients:

- 1 tablespoon olive oil
- 1 clove garlic, chopped
- ½ teaspoon ground cumin
- ½ teaspoon ground coriander
- A large pinch ground allspice
- 1 small onion, chopped
- ½ tablespoons chipotle chili in adobo sauce
- 1 teaspoon swerve or erythritol
- 2 cups broth
- 1 cup pumpkin puree
- ¼ cup heavy cream
- Salt to taste
- Pepper to taste
- 1 teaspoon red wine vinegar
- Sour cream to garnish

Method:

1. Place a saucepan over medium flame and add oil. When the oil is heated, add onions and garlic and sauté until translucent.
2. Add cumin, coriander, allspice, pepper, swerve and chipotle chili and cook for a couple of minutes.
3. Stir in pumpkin puree and broth and let it simmer for 5 minutes.

4. Blend with an immersion blender until smooth.
5. Add rest of the ingredients and stir. Simmer for 3-4 minutes.
6. Ladle into soup bowls. Drizzle some sour cream on top and serve.

Spicy Tomato and Blue Cheese Soup

Serves: 2-3

Ingredients:

- 1 tablespoon olive oil
- 1 small red onion, minced
- 14 ounces canned tomatoes with its juice
- 6 tablespoons heavy cream
- A handful fresh oregano, chopped
- Greek yogurt to garnish
- 1 sprig oregano
- Salt to taste
- Pepper to taste
- 2 cloves garlic, peeled, sliced
- ¾ cup stock
- 1 tablespoons sriracha sauce
- ¼ cup Roth Kase Buttermilk Blue cheese
- Hot sauce to garnish

Method:

1. Place a skillet over medium heat. Add oil. When the oil is heated, add onions and a large pinch salt. Sauté until translucent.
2. Add garlic and cook for a couple of minutes.
3. Stir in the tomatoes and stock. Add oregano sprig, cream, fresh oregano and sriracha sauce and let it simmer for a while. Turn off the heat.
4. Discard the oregano sprig. Cool for a while.

5. Transfer into a blender and blend until smooth. Pass the soup through a fine wire mesh strainer into a saucepan.
6. Taste and adjust the seasonings if required. Heat thoroughly.
7. Ladle into soup bowls. Spoon yogurt on top. Drizzle hot sauce and serve.

Buffalo Ranch Chicken Soup

Serves: 6

Ingredients:

- 2 cups chicken breast, skinless, boneless
- 2 tablespoons ranch dressing
- A little olive oil
- 1 small yellow onion, chopped
- 4 ounces cream cheese
- 4 cups chicken broth
- 1 tablespoon hot sauce
- 1 stalk celery, chopped
- 3 tablespoons salted butter
- ½ cup heavy whipping cream
- 3 slices bacon
- A handful parsley, chopped, to serve

Method:

1. Place a skillet over medium heat. Add a little olive oil. When the oil is heated, add chicken and cook until brown. Flip sides and cook the other side too. Add about a cup of water and cook the chicken until tender. Add more water if required.
2. Turn off the heat. When cool enough to handle, shred the chicken with a pair of forks and set aside.
3. Place the skillet back over heat. Add bacon and cook until crisp.

4. Meanwhile, add rest of the ingredients into a saucepan. Place the saucepan over medium heat. Let it heat.
5. Add chicken and bacon and simmer for 6-8 minutes.
6. Ladle into soup bowls. Garnish with parsley and serve.

Creamy Leek and Salmon Soup

Serves: 2 large servings

Ingredients:

- 1 tablespoon avocado oil
- 2 cloves garlic, minced
- 1 teaspoon dried thyme
- 1 cup coconut milk
- 2 leeks, trimmed, cut into half moons
- 3 cups chicken broth or seafood broth
- ½ pound salmon, cut into bite size pieces, thaw if frozen
- Salt to taste
- Pepper to taste

Method:

1. Place a Dutch oven or soup pot over medium low heat. When the oil is heated, add garlic and leeks and sauté until translucent.
2. Stir in stock and thyme. Let it simmer for 8-10 minutes.
3. Add salt, pepper, salmon and coconut milk. Cook until the fish turns opaque.
4. Ladle into soup bowls and serve.

Southwestern Pork Stew

Serves: 4

Ingredients:

- 1 tablespoon avocado oil
- 2 cups chicken broth
- ¾ cup rutabaga, peeled, cubed
- 1 clove garlic, sliced
- ¾ teaspoon dried oregano
- ¼ teaspoon ground cumin
- 3 lime wedges
- 1 ¼ pounds pork chops, boneless
- 7.5 ounces canned diced tomato
- 1 small onion, chopped
- ½ tablespoon chili powder
- ½ teaspoon kosher salt or to taste
- ¼ teaspoon pepper powder or to taste

Method:

1. Add all the ingredients into a soup pot. Mix well.
2. Place over low heat. Cook until pork is tender.
3. Remove pork with a slotted spoon and place on your cutting board.
4. When cool enough to handle, shred the pork and add it back into the pot.
5. Simmer for some more time.
6. Ladle into bowls and serve with lime wedges.

Chapter 9: Ketogenic Dinner Recipes

Keto Pizza

Serves: 4

Ingredients:

For crust:

- 12 ounces cheese like mozzarella cheese or provolone cheese
- 2 eggs

For topping:

- 1 ½ tablespoons tomato paste
- 2 ounces cheese, shredded
- ½ teaspoon dried oregano
- Olives, sliced
- ¾ ounce pepperoni slices

For serving:

- 2.75 ounces leafy greens
- Salt to taste
- Pepper to taste
- 2 tablespoons olive oil

Method:

1. Add eggs into a bowl. Whisk well. Add cheese and stir.

2. Line a baking sheet with parchment paper. Pour the egg mixture into the baking sheet.
3. Bake in a preheated oven at 400° F for 15 minutes or until golden brown.
4. Remove from the oven and cool for a few minutes.
5. Increase the temperature of the oven to 450° F.
6. Layer the crust with tomato paste. Sprinkle oregano and cheese.
7. Top with pepperoni and olive slices.
8. Bake for 5-10 minutes.
9. Serve with a keto friendly salad of your choice.

Pesto Chicken Casserole with Feta Cheese and Olives

Serves: 6

Ingredients:

- 2 ¼ pounds chicken thighs or chicken breasts, chopped into pieces
- 4.5 ounces red or green pesto
- ¾ cup pitted olives
- 2 cloves garlic, minced
- 3 ounces butter, for frying
- 2 ¼ cups heavy whipping cream
- 4 ounces feta cheese, chopped
- Salt to taste
- Pepper to taste

To serve:

- 8 ounces leafy greens
- Salt to taste
- Pepper to taste
- 6 tablespoons olive oil

Method:

1. Place a skillet over medium heat. Add butter. When butter melts, sprinkle salt and pepper over the chicken and place chicken in the skillet. Cook until golden brown.
2. Transfer into a greased baking dish.

3. Add pesto and cream into a bowl and mix well. Pour over the chicken. Add olives, garlic and feta cheese and stir.
4. Bake in a preheated oven at 400° F for 15 minutes or until light brown.

Meat Pie

Serves: 3

Ingredients:

- 1 medium onion, finely chopped
- 1 tablespoon olive oil
- Salt to taste
- Pepper to taste
- 2 tablespoons tomato paste or ajvar relish
- 1 clove garlic, minced
- ¾ pound ground lamb or beef
- ½ tablespoon dried herbs of your choice
- ¼ cup water

For pie crust:

- 2 tablespoons coconut flour
- 6 tablespoons almond flour
- 2 tablespoons sesame seeds
- A pinch salt
- 1 small egg
- ½ teaspoon baking powder
- 1 ½ tablespoons olive oil or coconut oil or butter
- ½ tablespoon ground psyllium husk powder
- 2 tablespoons water

For topping:

- 3.5 ounces cheese, shredded
- 4 ounces cottage cheese

Method:

1. Place a skillet over medium heat. Add oil. When oil is heated, add onions and garlic and sauté until translucent.
2. Stir in meat and sauté until brown. Add oregano, salt and pepper and mix well.
3. Add tomato paste and water and mix well.
4. Reduce heat to low heat and simmer for 10-15 minutes.
5. Meanwhile, make the crust as follows: Add all the ingredients into a bowl and mix into a dough. Alternately, you can use a food processor to make the dough.
6. Grease a small springform pan of about 6 inches with a little butter. Place a sheet of parchment paper in the pan.
7. Spread the dough in the pan. Press it well on to the bottom as well as the sides of the pan.
8. Bake in a preheated oven at 350° F for 10-15 minutes.
9. Spread the meat mixture on the crust. Mix together cottage cheese and shredded cheese in a bowl and spread over the meat.
10. Bake until the top is golden brown in color.
11. Serve with a green salad.

Sausage with Creamed Green Cabbage

Serves: 2

Ingredients:

For fried chorizo:

- 1 tablespoon butter to fry
- ¾ pound chorizo or any other sausage

Creamed green cabbage:

- ¾ pound green cabbage
- 10 tablespoons heavy whipping cream
- ¼ cup fresh parsley, finely chopped
- A handful fresh parsley, chopped
- 1 ounce butter
- Salt to taste
- Pepper to taste
- ½ teaspoon lemon zest, grated

Method:

1. Cook the chorizo following the instructions.
2. Place a skillet over medium heat. Add butter. When butter melts, add cabbage and sauté until golden brown.
3. Add cream and stir. When it begins to boil, lower heat and let it simmer for 5-6 minutes.
4. Add salt and pepper.
5. Garnish with parsley and lemon zest and serve.

Turkey with Cream Cheese Sauce

Serves: 6

Ingredients:

- 2 ¼ pounds turkey breast
- 3 cups crème fraiche or heavy whipping cream
- Salt to taste
- Pepper to taste
- 1 ½ tablespoons tamari sauce
- 3 tablespoons butter
- 7.5 ounces cream cheese
- ¾ cup small capers

Method:

1. Place a large ovenproof pan over medium flame and add half the butter. When butter melts, sprinkle salt and pepper over the turkey and place the turkey in the skillet. Cook until golden brown. Turn off the heat.
2. Transfer the pan into the oven.
3. Bake in a preheated oven at 350° F until turkey is cooked.
4. Remove the turkey from the oven and place on a plate. Cover the turkey with foil and let it rest for a while.
5. Add the turkey drippings into a saucepan. Add crème fraiche or heavy whipping cream into it and mix well.

6. Place over low heat and simmer until thick. Add tamari, salt and pepper and mix well.
7. Place another pan over medium flame and add remaining butter. When butter melts, add capers and cook until crisp.
8. Serve turkey with sauce and capers.

Spaghetti Squash Lasagna with Meat Casserole

Serves: 4

Ingredients:

- 1 small spaghetti squash, cooked
- ¼ cup parmesan cheese
- ½ pound beef
- ½ cup mozzarella cheese
- ¾ cup ricotta cheese
- 1 medium egg
- ¾ cup keto friendly spaghetti squash

Method:

1. Using a spoon scoop the squash and place in a kitchen towel. Wring the towel to squeeze out excess moisture from the squash.
2. Spread on the bottom of a square baking dish of about 6 inches. Spread it evenly.
3. Add ricotta cheese, Parmesan cheese and egg into a bowl. Spread it over the squash.
4. Spread meat over the ricotta layer. Spread spaghetti sauce over it.
5. Sprinkle mozzarella cheese on top.
6. Bake in a preheated oven at 350° F for about 20 minutes or until brown.

Smoked Salmon Plate

Serves: 4

Ingredients:

- 1 ½ pounds smoked salmon
- 4 ounces baby spinach
- Lime wedges to serve, optional
- 2 cups keto friendly mayonnaise
- 2 tablespoons olive oil
- Salt to taste
- Pepper to taste

Method:

1. Add salmon, spinach and mayonnaise into a bowl and fold gently.
2. Add salt and pepper and fold gently.
3. Divide among 4 plates. Drizzle oil and serve with lemon wedges.

Chapter 10: Ketogenic Side Dish Recipes

Creamy Spaghetti Squash Ricotta

Serves: 8

Ingredients:

- 2 spaghetti squash, halved, deseeded
- 1 teaspoon garlic powder
- 2 tablespoons olive oil
- 2 cups plain, full fat Greek yogurt
- 4 tablespoons fresh basil or parsley, chopped
- 6 tablespoons parmesan cheese, shredded
- ¾ cup + 2 tablespoons ricotta cheese
- 2 teaspoons dried oregano
- 2 eggs
- Salt to taste
- Pepper to taste

Method:

1. Spray the cut part of the spaghetti squash with cooking spray.
2. Place it on a baking sheet with the cut side down. Pour a little water around the spaghetti squash.
3. Bake in a preheated oven at 375° F for about 40-50 minutes.

4. When done, using a fork, scrape the squash and add into a baking dish. Pour oil and mix well.
5. Lower the temperature of the oven to 350° F.
6. Add ricotta cheese, Parmesan cheese, yogurt, egg, oregano, garlic powder, salt, pepper and basil into a bowl and mix well.
7. Transfer into the baking dish. Mix until well combined.
8. Bake for 20-30 minutes.

Goat Cheese Cauliflower Bake

Serves: 4

Ingredients:

- 1 large head cauliflower, cut into florets
- 1 medium onion, chopped
- 5 ounces goat's cheese, divided
- Salt to taste
- Pepper to taste
- 2 strips Hickory smoked bacon
- 2 teaspoons garlic, minced
- 2 tablespoons low fat cream cheese, softened
- 1 green onion, sliced, to garnish

Method:

1. Grease a small casserole dish with oil or butter.
2. Add cauliflower into a microwave safe bowl and microwave on high for 6-8 minutes or until tender.
3. Meanwhile, place a skillet over medium heat. Add bacon and cook until brown. Remove with a slotted spoon and place on a plate lined with paper towels. When cool enough to handle, chop into smaller pieces.
4. Add onion and garlic into the same skillet and cook until golden brown.
5. Add cauliflower, cream cheese, sautéed onion and half the goat's cheese into the food processor bowl and pulse until well combined.

6. Transfer into a bowl. Add bacon, salt and pepper and stir.
7. Transfer the cauliflower mixture into the prepared casserole dish.
8. Top with remaining goat's cheese.
9. Bake in a preheated oven at 400° F for about 20 minutes or until brown.
10. Sprinkle green onion on top and serve.

Cauliflower Steaks

Serves: 4

Ingredients:

- 2 cauliflowers
- 6 sun dried tomatoes, finely chopped
- 4 plum tomatoes, cored, quartered
- 6 tablespoons olive oil
- 1 teaspoon salt
- 1 cup black olives, pitted
- 6 cloves garlic, finely chopped
- 2 teaspoons lemon juice
- ¼ cup flat leaf parsley, chopped
- Pepper to taste

Method:

1. Place the cauliflowers on your cutting board and cut each into 4 large slices.
2. If any florets break away from the slice, chop it into fine pieces.
3. Add chopped cauliflower, parsley, salt, pepper, and olives, sun dried tomatoes, 2 tablespoons olive oil and lemon juice in a bowl and toss well.
4. Place a large skillet over medium heat. Add 4 tablespoons oil. When the oil is heated, place the cauliflower slices. (Cook in batches if required. If cooking in batches, add 1-2 tablespoons oil in each batch).

5. Cook until golden brown. Flip sides and cook the other side too.
6. Transfer on to a baking sheet that is lined with parchment paper. Place garlic and tomatoes alongside.
7. Bake in a preheated oven at 400° F for about 25 minutes or until brown.
8. When done, add the roasted garlic and tomato into a blender and blend until smooth.
9. Divide and pour the sauce into individual serving plates.
10. Place 2 cauliflower slices on each plate. Sprinkle sundried tomato mixture on top and serve.

Oven Fried Parmesan Zucchini Rounds

Serves: 6

Ingredients:

- 1 ½ large zucchinis, sliced into ½ cm thick slices
- 2 eggs, beaten
- ¼ teaspoon garlic powder or to taste
- A handful fresh parsley, chopped
- ¾ cup parmesan cheese, grated
- Olive oil cooking spray

Method:

1. Spray a large baking sheet with cooking spray.
2. Add Parmesan, parsley and garlic powder into a bowl and stir.
3. First, dip the zucchini slices in the egg. Shake to drop off excess egg. Next dredge in the Parmesan mixture and place on the baking sheet, in a single layer. Bake in batches if required.
4. Bake in a preheated oven at 425° F for about 20 minutes. Flip sides halfway through baking.
5. Bake until the top is golden brown.

Roasted Broccoli

Serves: 2

Ingredients:

- 2 cups broccoli florets
- 1 teaspoon Sriracha hot sauce
- ½ teaspoon lime juice
- 2 tablespoons keto friendly mayonnaise
- ½ teaspoon tamari

Method:

1. Steam the broccoli in the steaming equipment you have or in a microwave until it is crisp and tender as well.
2. Add rest of the ingredients into a baking dish and mix well. Add broccoli and toss well.
3. Broil for 3-4 minutes until slightly brown. Stir and continue broiling for a couple of minutes.
4. Serve hot.

Creamed Kale with Bacon and Walnuts

Serves: 5 (½ cup each)

Ingredients:

- 2 slices raw bacon, chopped
- 1 clove garlic, minced
- A large pinch ground nutmeg
- ½ cup mascarpone cheese
- Salt to taste
- Pepper to taste
- ½ tablespoon butter
- ¼ cup almond milk, unsweetened
- 5 cups raw kale leaves, discard hard stems and ribs, chopped
- 3 tablespoons parmesan cheese or Romano cheese, grated
- 2 tablespoons walnuts, chopped

Method:

1. Place a skillet over medium heat. Add bacon and cook until light brown. Do not make it crisp. Remove with a slotted spoon and set aside.
2. Add a pan over medium flame and add butter. When butter melts, add garlic and sauté until aromatic.
3. Stir in almond milk and nutmeg.

4. Add kale. Stir occasionally. Add mascarpone cheese and Parmesan cheese and mix until well combined. Add salt and pepper and stir.
5. Transfer into a casserole dish that is greased with a little butter or oil.
6. Bake in a preheated oven at 425° F for about 20 minutes.
7. Garnish with bacon and walnuts. Bake for 10 more minutes and serve.

Butternut Squash and Fennel Gratin

Serves: 5

Ingredients:

- 2 cups butternut squash slices, cut into ¼ inch thick slices
- 2 tablespoons salted butter + extra to grease
- 1 ½ cups fennel bulb, sliced
- 6 tablespoons almond milk, unsweetened
- 1 ounce blue cheese, grated
- 2 tablespoons heavy whipping cream
- Salt to taste
- Pepper to taste

Method:

1. Grease a small casserole dish with a little butter. Place a layer of squash. Sprinkle salt and pepper.
2. Place a layer of fennel over it. Sprinkle salt and pepper.
3. Add rest of the ingredients into a microwave safe bowl. Microwave on high for 1-2 minutes until it melts. You can also heat in a saucepan.
4. Pour over the vegetable layers in the dish.
5. Cover the dish with foil, loosely.
6. Bake in a preheated oven at 350° F for about 40-60 minutes or until tender and light brown on top.
7. When done, let it rest for 10 minutes.

8. Serve.

Chapter 11: Ketogenic Dessert Recipes

Pumpkin Spices Chocolate Slab

Serves: 24

Ingredients:

- 8 pumpkin spiced collagen bars, chopped
- 2 cups cocoa powder, unsweetened
- 1 tablespoon ghee
- Swerve or stevia to taste
- ½ teaspoon vanilla powder
- ½ cup cacao butter
- ¼ teaspoon salt

Method:

1. Place a small saucepan over low heat. Add ghee and cacao butter. Let it melt. Stir occasionally.
2. Stir in the cocoa, vanilla, swerve and salt until well combined.
3. Place a sheet of parchment paper in a dish.
4. Pour the chocolate mixture in the dish.
5. Top with spiced collagen bars. Chill for a couple of hours until firm.
6. Chop into 24 equal squares and serve.
7. Leftovers can be stored in an airtight container in the refrigerator.

Easy Raspberry Coconut Bar Fat Bombs

Serves: 24

Ingredients:

- 1 cup freeze dried raspberries
- 1 cup coconut oil
- ½ cup powdered swerve sweetener
- 1 cup coconut butter
- 1 cup shredded coconut, unsweetened

Method:

1. Take a square pan and line with parchment paper. Set aside.
2. Add freeze-dried raspberries into a coffee grinder or spice grinder. Process until it is powdered fine.
3. Place a saucepan over medium flame and add coconut butter, coconut oil, shredded coconut and swerve. Stir frequently until the mixture is well combined. Turn off the heat.
4. Spoon half the mixture into the prepared pan. To the other half of the mixture, add the raspberry powder and mix well.
5. Now spoon the raspberry mixture over the coconut layer. Take a blunt knife and swirl the mixture.
6. Freeze for a couple of hours.

7. Cut into 24 equal pieces and serve. Leftovers can be stored in an airtight container in the refrigerator.

Low Carb Chocolate Mint Pudding

Serves: 8

Ingredients:

- 3 cups full fat coconut milk or heavy cream
- 7 tablespoons cocoa powder, unsweetened
- 4 tablespoons coconut oil
- ½ teaspoon mint extract
- 6 tablespoons cold water
- 2 yolks, beaten
- 1 cup erythritol
- ½ teaspoon gluten free vanilla extract
- 2 tablespoons unflavored gelatin

Optional toppings:

- A handful dark chocolate chips, unsweetened
- 4 tablespoons heavy whipped cream or coconut cream
- Stevia drops to taste

Method:

1. Add cold water into a bowl. Add gelatin and whisk until well combined. Set aside for a while.
2. Place a saucepan over medium heat.
3. Add rest of the ingredients and whisk constantly all the while until well combined.

4. Lower heat and whisk in the gelatin water. Whisk constantly until well combined. Turn off the heat. Cool for a while.
5. Pour into 8 custard cups. Chill for a few hours until set.
6. Top with whipped cream and chocolate chips if using and serve.

Strawberry Mousse

Serves: 12

Ingredients:

- 3 cups firm tofu, drained, crumbled
- 3 cups strawberries, sliced + extra to garnish
- Erythritol or stevia to taste
- Dark chocolate, unsweetened, shaved to garnish

Method:

1. Blend the strawberries in a blender until smooth. Add tofu and sweetener and blend until smooth. Add a tablespoon of milk if desired while blending
2. Transfer into 12 dessert bowls and refrigerate for a few hours before serving.

Chocolate Chip Cookies

Serves: 9

Ingredients:

For dry ingredients:

- 1 ¼ cups almond flour
- ¼ teaspoon baking soda
- ¼ teaspoon salt
- ¼ cup erythritol

For wet ingredients:

- 2 tablespoons walnuts, chopped
- 1 large egg
- ¼ cup dark chocolate chips
- ¼ cup unsalted butter, melted
- ½ tablespoon vanilla extract

Method:

1. Add all the dry ingredients into a bowl and mix well.
2. Add all the wet ingredients into another bowl and mix until well combined.
3. Pour the wet ingredients into the bowl of dry ingredients and mix into a dough.
4. Divide the mixture into 9 equal portions and shape into cookies.
5. Place on a baking sheet that is lined with parchment paper.

6. Bake in a preheated oven at 350° F for about 8-10 minutes or until the edges are golden brown in color.
7. Remove the baking sheet from the oven and place on a cooling rack to cool completely.
8. Serve. Leftovers can be stored in an airtight container.

Hot Chocolate Ice Cream

Serves: 6

- 1 can (14 ounces) canned coconut milk, chilled
- 1 tablespoons cocoa powder
- 2 scoops chocolate protein powder, unsweetened
- 1 tablespoon swerve or erythritol

Method:

1. Add the coconut milk into a blender. Blend until smooth.
2. Add rest of the ingredients and blend again until well combined.
3. Pour into a chilled freezer safe pan. Freeze for a couple of hours until firm.
4. Stir the ice cream after an hour.
5. Scoop into bowls and serve.

Berry Berry Ambrosia

Serves: 12 small servings

Ingredients:

- 1 ½ cups sugar free cherry jello
- ½ cup heavy cream
- ½ teaspoon vanilla extract
- 1 ½ cups berries, chopped
- 3 ounces cream, cut into cubes, at room temperature
- 2 packets Splenda naturals or ½ tablespoon stevia blend

Method:

1. Add heavy cream into a chilled bowl and beat with a hand mixer until peaks are formed.
2. Add swerve and vanilla and whisk again.
3. Add cream cheese and whisk until well combined.
4. Add berries and jello. Fold gently. Chill if desired.
5. Serve.

Chapter 12: 2 Weeks Meal Plan

Day 1

Breakfast - Ultimate Breakfast Roll Ups

Lunch - Broccoli Cheddar Soup

Snack - Sesame Crisp Bread

Dinner - Smoked Salmon Plate

Desserts - Pumpkin Spices Chocolate Slab

Day 2

Breakfast - Berry Smoothie

Lunch - High Fat Hamburger Soup

Snack - Salad Sandwiches

Dinner - Roasted Broccoli

Desserts - Easy Raspberry Coconut Bar Fat Bombs

Day 3

Breakfast - 3 Cheese Quiche Stuffed Peppers

Lunch - Spicy Tomato and Blue Cheese Soup

Snack - Cheese Chips

Dinner - Creamy Spaghetti Squash Ricotta

Desserts - Low Carb Chocolate Mint Pudding

Day 4

Breakfast - Vanilla Smoothie

Lunch - Southwestern Pork Stew

Snack - Prosciutto Wrapped Mozzarella

Dinner - Spaghetti Squash Lasagna with Meat Casserole

Desserts - Strawberry Mousse

Day 5

Breakfast - Spinach Herb and Feta Wraps

Lunch - Pesto Chicken Casserole with Feta Cheese and Olives

Snack - Cheese Meatballs

Dinner - Creamy Leek and Salmon Soup

Desserts - Hot Chocolate Ice Cream

Day 6

Breakfast - Raspberry Avocado Smoothie

Lunch - Smoked Salmon Plate

Snack - Cheese Puffs

Dinner - Pumpkin Chipotle Soup

Desserts - Chocolate Chip Cookies

Day 7

Breakfast - Avocado Bacon Muffins

Lunch - Sausage with Creamed Green Cabbage

Snack - Keto Apple Slaw

Dinner - Spaghetti Squash Lasagna with Meat Casserole

Desserts - Berry Berry Ambrosia

Day 8

Breakfast - Green Lemon Smoothie

Lunch - Creamed Kale with Bacon and Walnuts

Snack - Sesame Crisp Bread

Dinner - Creamy Spaghetti Squash Ricotta

Desserts - Pumpkin Spices Chocolate Slab

Day 9

Breakfast - Frozen Peppermint Hot Chocolate

Lunch - Spaghetti Squash Lasagna with Meat Casserole

Snack - Chicken and Berry Summer Salad

Dinner - Oven Fried Parmesan Zucchini Rounds

Desserts - Easy Raspberry Coconut Bar Fat Bombs

Day 10

Breakfast - French toast Muffin

Lunch - Goat Cheese Cauliflower Bake

Snack - Chicken Salad Eggs

Dinner - Meat Pie

Desserts - Low Carb Chocolate Mint Pudding

Day 11

Breakfast - Mexican Chocolate Shake

Lunch - Butternut Squash and Fennel Gratin

Snack - Prosciutto Wrapped Mozzarella

Dinner - Butternut Squash and Fennel Gratin

Desserts - Strawberry Mousse

Day 12

Breakfast - Mini Pancake Donuts

Lunch - Cauliflower Steaks

Snack - Caesar Salad

Dinner - Buffalo Ranch Chicken Soup

Desserts - Hot Chocolate Ice Cream

Day 13

Breakfast - Pumpkin Smoothie

Lunch - Turkey with Cream Cheese Sauce

Snack - Avocado, Bacon and Goat's Cheese Salad

Dinner - Sausage with Creamed Green Cabbage

Desserts - Chocolate Chip Cookies

Day 14

Breakfast - Breakfast Stack

Lunch - Roasted Broccoli

Snack - Warm Kale Salad

Dinner - Meat Pie

Desserts - Berry Berry Ambrosia

Conclusion

On that note, we have come to the end of this book. I would once again like to thank you for purchasing this book!

I trust you had an informative read and are all pumped up to venture into the ketogenic diet armed with all the information and recipes compiled into this book just for you!

People have always struggled to figure out which diet to opt for and how – since there are so many and each comes with its own specifications and set of benefits. Everyone has their own reason to take an interest in the ketogenic diet and then be completely besotted by everything the diet offers – from the health benefits to the interesting choice of foods you get to experience and experiment when you are on the ketogenic diet.

You can probably hear your kitchen calling out to you to try out all the amazing recipes you just read about! Well – all the best with discovering a whole new culinary world and experiences.

Finally, if you enjoyed this book, would you be kind enough to leave a review for this book on Amazon?

Click here to leave a review for this book on Amazon!

https://www.amazon.com/dp/B079QZZ5C8/ref=sr_1_126?s=digital-text&ie=UTF8&qid=1518373208&sr=1-126&keywords=ketogenic+diet

Thank you and good luck!

28057644R00063

Printed in Great Britain
by Amazon